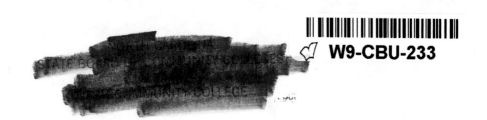
W9-CBU-233

Body Blues: Weight and Depression

Body Blues:
Weight and Depression

Laura Weeldreyer

The Rosen Publishing Group/New York

The Teen Health
Library of
Eating Disorder
Prevention

For Tina

I'd like to thank the following people for their wisdom, support, and encouragment: Alice Halle and Tahira Archer (my junior editors), Caitlin Cornwell, Michele Drohan, Doug Fireside, Eileen O'Brien, Colleen Pierre, R.D., and friends, family and coworkers too numerous to list.

Published in 1998 by The Rosen Publishing Group, Inc.
29 East 21st Street, New York, NY 10010

Copyright © 1998 by The Rosen Publishing Group, Inc.

First Edition

Library of Congress Cataloging-in-Publication Data

Weeldreyer, Laura.
    Body blues: weight and depression / by Laura Weeldreyer.
    p. cm. — (The teen health library of eating disorder prevention)
    Includes index.
    ISBN 0-8239-2761-X
    1. Body weight—Psychological aspects. 2. Eating disorders—Psychological aspects.
3. Eating disorders—Popular works. 4. Eating disorders in adolescence—Popular works.
5. Depression, Mental—Nutritional aspects. 6. Depression, Mental—Popular works.
7. Depression in adolescence—popular works. 8. Weight loss—Psychological aspects.
9. Body image—Popular works. I. Title. II. Series.
RC552.025W44 1998
616.85'26'0019—dc21   98-20226
                                                                                            CIP
                                                                                             AC

Manufactured in the United States of America

Contents

Introduction

What do you see when you look in the mirror? Are you satisfied with your appearance? Do you feel sad and angry at yourself because you think you're fat or ugly? Do you wish you could change your looks? Do you criticize yourself a lot? Are there parts of your body you really dislike?

Most people worry about their appearance and their weight at some point in their lives. For some people, worrying about how they look and battling with food is a part of every day. It's not unusual to hear people say, "I wish I could lose ten pounds," or "I would do anything to look like a model." Are similar feelings keeping you from enjoying life? Do you have an inner critic that is constantly putting you down for the way you look? Do you spend a large part of every day planning what and when you will eat and then punishing yourself for what you do eat? If so, you may be suffering from the body blues, or feelings of depression as a result of your preoccupation with your appearance.

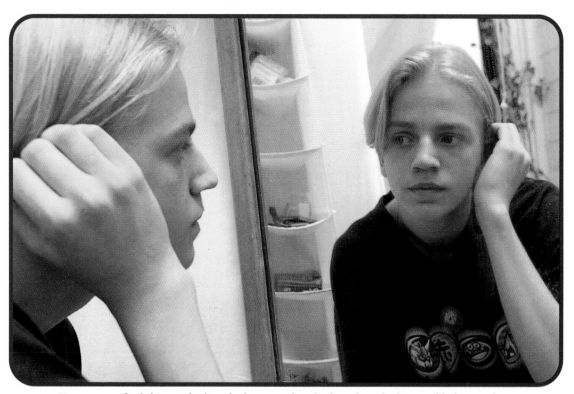

Many teens feel dissatisfied with the way they look and wish they could change their appearance.

The body blues—negative thinking about your body and your appearance that affects the way you feel about your whole self—may be contributing to your feelings of depression. You may think that being fat or thin determines whether you are smart or stupid, whether you will have friends, and even whether you are a success or failure in life. Many people are convinced that looking "good" is the same as being a good person. You may think that you have to look a certain way to be liked and accepted.

All of us have our own relationships with food. These relationships range from healthy ("Food is fuel for my body, and a healthy diet means a happier, stronger me") to unhealthy ("Food is my enemy, so I skip meals or I eat too much and feel guilty"). Food is neither good nor bad, but we may see it that way because of society's vision of how we should look, our feelings about how we look, and how we think food affects our appearance.

When people are addicted to drugs or cigarettes, there are many programs to help them quit and conquer their addictions. Food is different. We cannot give up food completely because we need it to live. That is one reason why it is important to develop a healthy relationship with food.

Teenage girls are most at risk of suffering from depression linked to feelings about their weight. Researchers have found that young girls care more than boys do about what other people think of them and about being liked—which they believe is linked to whether they are pretty or ugly, thin or fat. This is not surprising considering that our society sends a strong message to young girls about the importance of being thin and beautiful.

Television, movies, magazines, and advertisements surround us with unrealistic images of men and women. It is easy to believe that beauty and success or happiness are strongly connected. What may surprise you is that the result of this societal pressure is depression for many teenagers. Doctors have found that depression in teenage girls has a lot to do with how unhappy they are about their weight. Young people are beginning to worry about their weight at earlier and earlier ages. A survey of 500 ten-year-old girls in San Francisco showed that 405 of them had been on a diet at least once—before they had reached the fourth grade.

Although we may all suffer from a touch of the body blues at some point in our lives, some of us need help in dealing with the negative feelings that arise as a result of depression. Depression can also lead to eating disorders, and eating disorders can lead to further depression. Teenagers can become trapped in this cycle without realizing the serious risks they are posing to their mental and physical health. Hopefully you are reading this book before you reach such a serious point.

This book will offer some suggestions on how to help yourself or someone you know, and, if needed, how to find outside help. Most important, this book will give you the information you need to break the cycle of depression and negative thoughts and to take control of your life.

The Body Blues

1

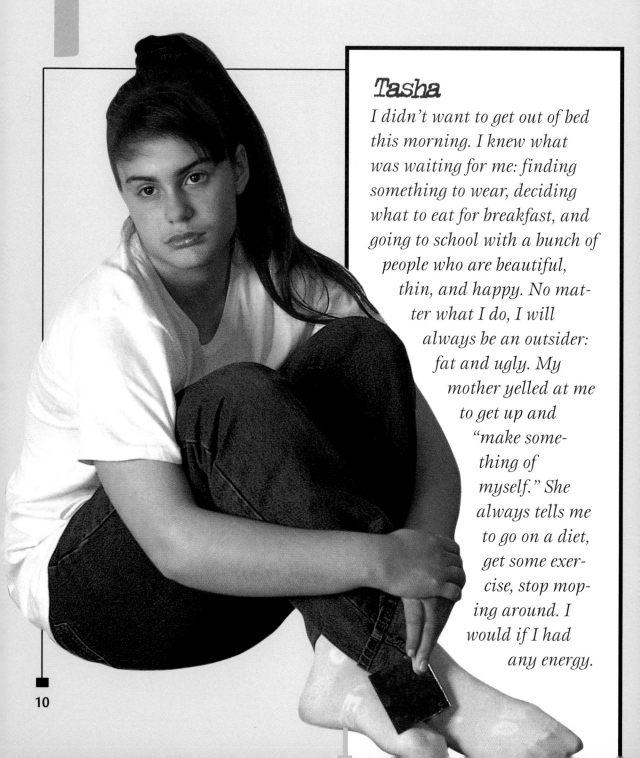

Tasha

I didn't want to get out of bed this morning. I knew what was waiting for me: finding something to wear, deciding what to eat for breakfast, and going to school with a bunch of people who are beautiful, thin, and happy. No matter what I do, I will always be an outsider: fat and ugly. My mother yelled at me to get up and "make something of myself." She always tells me to go on a diet, get some exercise, stop moping around. I would if I had any energy.

But what's the point? Some people were born to be beautiful. I wasn't. That's never going to change.

What Are the Body Blues?

You will not find "body blues" in a dictionary, and it is not a medical term. However, having the body blues is a reality for many teens. In this book, body blues refers to negative thoughts and feelings about yourself—anger, sadness, and depression— because of the way you look. A lot of people do not accept themselves or like themselves. Some believe that they are bad or failures because of how they look. Appearance, for many, becomes the most important way of defining themselves.

Body Image

How you perceive yourself, and how comfortable or satisfied you are with your appearance and weight, is called your body image. Our body image plays a big role in how we think of ourselves. A negative body image can lead to depression and even to eating disorders, such as anorexia nervosa and bulimia nervosa.

Having a distorted body image is like looking in a funhouse mirror: You see yourself as heavier, shorter, taller, or thinner than you really are.

Where does your body image come from? We live in a society that places a high value on appearance.

Teenagers face pressures from several sources: parents, friends, and the media (television, movies, magazines). We develop our body image as a response to the influences we experience. There is enormous pressure to be thin and attractive in our culture. There is no link between being smart, talented, or interesting and being attractive, although society may send the opposite message.

Self-Esteem

Your self-esteem and your identity can become tied up with how you look. Positive self-esteem flows from feelings of pride in who you are and what you do. Negative self-esteem is often the painful result of judging yourself as inadequate. Until the age of twenty, approval from our family, our school, and our peers is the strongest influence on our self-esteem. Each new stage of life and each new challenge present opportunities to enhance your self-esteem or reverse a negative outlook.

Using your body image to define yourself can be damaging to your self-esteem. People are more than just what they look like on the outside. Sometimes we can change what we don't like about our appearance, and sometimes we can't. Becoming fixated on your appearance may keep you from enjoying life, experiencing new things, and learning more about yourself.

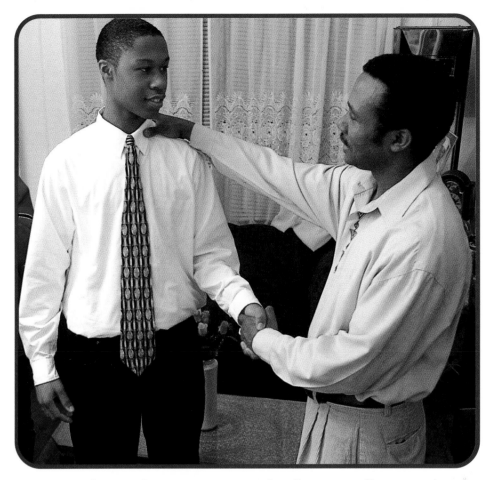

Praise and support from our parents strongly influence our self-esteem and body image as we grow up.

Tasha

I am writing this while all my friends are at Paul's swim party. I couldn't go because there is no way I will wear a bathing suit in front of my friends. If they saw how fat I really am, they wouldn't want to be friends with me. I hate summer! I don't want to wear shorts or sleeveless shirts or bathing suits. I am going to hide out until fall. My friends are angry at me for not going to the party, but they just don't understand.

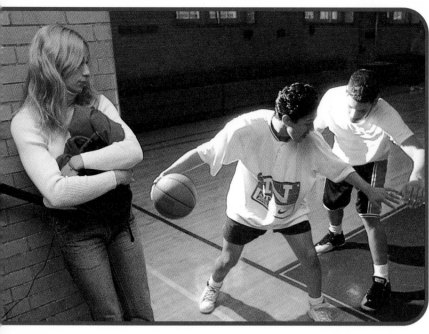

Some teens have such a negative body image that it prevents them from engaging in sports or other group activities with their friends.

Experts say the healthiest self-esteem comes from within. Many books and guides offer advice on raising your self-esteem by finding the best of yourself and cultivating a sense of your own value. It is normal to experience periods of low self-esteem. However, for some people, low self-esteem can be the first step toward depression.

What Is Depression?

We all have feelings of depression at one time or another. Certain events or situations in our lives can make us feel sad and lonely. But when these feelings last a long time and affect your daily life, you may be suffering from depression. Frequent symptoms of depression include:

- ❑ lack of motivation
- ❑ trouble sleeping

❏ constant fatigue
❏ withdrawal from friends
❏ feeling angry and/or sad all the time
❏ inability to concentrate
❏ poor memory
❏ unexplained headaches, backaches, or
  stomach pains
❏ inconsistencies in eating
❏ feelings of worthlessness

Mild depression is very common and is experienced by many of us. Serious depression is not as common, but it does affect one in five people at some time in life. Women are twice as likely as men to be affected by depression.

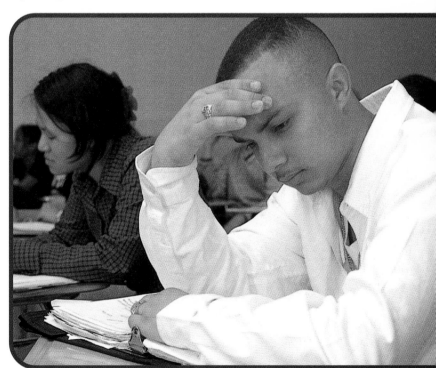

Having trouble concentrating is a common symptom of depression. This can cause difficulties at home and at school.

Depression is often misunderstood. We tell ourselves, or others tell us, to cheer up and "get over it." When we, or others, deny our feelings, we suffer. Depression should be taken seriously. Confirming and recognizing our feelings are the first step toward treating depression. Yet, because it often goes unrecognized, depression causes a lot of unnecessary suffering.

The Connection Between Depression and Weight

Depression can make us feel exhausted, worthless, and hopeless. Such negative thoughts and feelings can make some of us feel like giving up. But it's important to realize that these negative views are a part of the depression and do not actually reflect our situation. A recent study at Princeton University suggests that teenage depression in girls is related to their feelings about their weight. However, depression often distorts the girls' body image. The girls in the study fixated on what they saw as their physical shortcomings. They rated their appearance much lower than their peers rated it.

More and more doctors believe there is a link between depression and eating disorders. The two problems share many symptoms. Now doctors believe there may be some common ways of treating both illnesses. For years doctors have assumed that depression was a symptom of a patient's eating disorder. Now

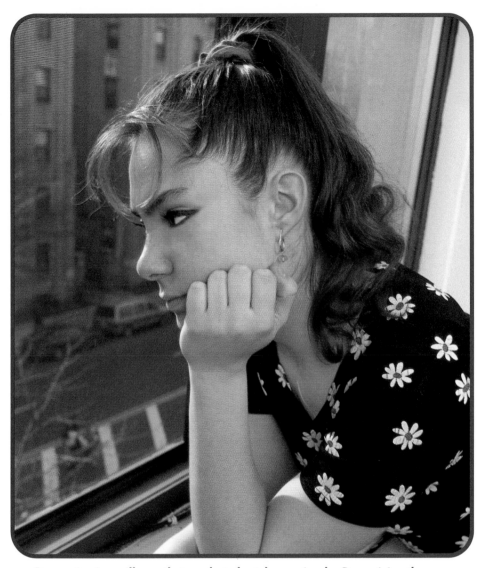

Depression is an illness that needs to be taken seriously. Recognizing the symptoms is the first step toward getting help.

they are considering the possibility that the eating disorder is a symptom of a patient's depression.

Treating Depression and Eating Disorders

The parts of the brain that regulate our emotional

lives are interconnected with the parts that regulate our eating. Antidepressants are medications that are commonly used to treat depression. Recently doctors have had some success using those same medications to treat patients suffering from eating disorders.

Studies have shown that antidepressants, such as Prozac, can significantly reduce the urge to overeat, restore a normal appetite function, and improve the motivation and commitment to follow a healthy lifestyle. These are all very valuable results given that eating disorders can be life-threatening. Many doctors now recommend screening of eating disorder patients for depression to see if they might benefit from Prozac or another antidepressant.

Jeanna

Every time I look in the mirror, I feel like crying. I don't know who that ugly fat face belongs to, and then I realize it's me. I look like a monster. When I see my reflection, I can't stop putting myself down. I think about my weight all the time, but I don't know what to do about it. I feel like no one will ever like me. All they will ever see is my fat body—I have to find a way out.

It doesn't matter which comes first: Depression may lead to a negative body image, or a negative body image may lead to being depressed. Depression is treatable, and a negative body image can be overcome. Whichever comes first, it is clear that there is a direct relationship between our feelings about our weight and appearance and feelings of depression.

The Unreal Ideal

2

Michael

This morning I was planning to ask Amy out on a date for this weekend. I was so nervous, but I was ready to do it. Then I heard her talking about the new Arnold Schwarzenegger movie and how cute and buff Arnold is. How can I compete with that? I'm just a regular guy, and now I feel like that's not enough.

Cultural Influences

We live in a world where skinny models are idolized and 60 percent of high school girls want to lose weight, according to a *Seventeen* magazine study. From fashion magazines and television to movies and music videos, the media portray unrealistic images of women's and men's bodies. For most people, trying to achieve the body shapes seen in the media is impossible and unhealthy. As we grow, our bodies mature. For young people this means growing larger and taller, and filling out in various areas of the body. This growth may be welcomed in men, but the media send us messages that women should stay skinny.

These messages are hard to ignore, but it's important not to compare yourself to what the media say is "ideal." Think about how you look and how you feel as an individual. Value yourself for qualities that count. It's important to realize that models do not represent real bodies. Look at real people in real pictures and in real situations. Then look carefully at pictures of models in magazines: What you see is the product of hours of professional attention from hairdressers and makeup artists and often the result of airbrushing of the photo. No one can compete with that in everyday life!

In our society, the media have promoted the idea that physical perfection is important and that our appearance somehow defines what kind of people we are. The message is that happiness, popularity, and success are all linked to how we look. We can blame the media for making a single look—impossible for most people to achieve—the ideal. But we do not have to accept that our looks measure our self-worth. You can't weigh your worth on a scale.

The Truth About Weight Charts

The perfect weight for you cannot be determined by a schedule or chart. Some of us have had the unpleasant experience of being weighed at the doctor's office and hearing a lecture that our weight is too high for our height according to a chart on the wall. This is an outdated way of thinking. Research suggests that a person's weight is not an accurate picture of the person's health. The number on the scale does not give enough information and can be misleading. If you exercise and increase muscle mass, your weight will actually go up, not down. But seeing that you have gained weight may discourage you from continuing your exercise program. Scales don't give us a full picture of what's happening inside our bodies.

What Do Genes Have to Do with It?

Body size, bone structure, weight, and height are largely determined by genetics. Our parents have more to do with our body size than our diets do. Our genes shape our bodies, both inside and out, and make it extremely difficult, and unhealthy, to reshape ourselves into another body size. Some doctors believe

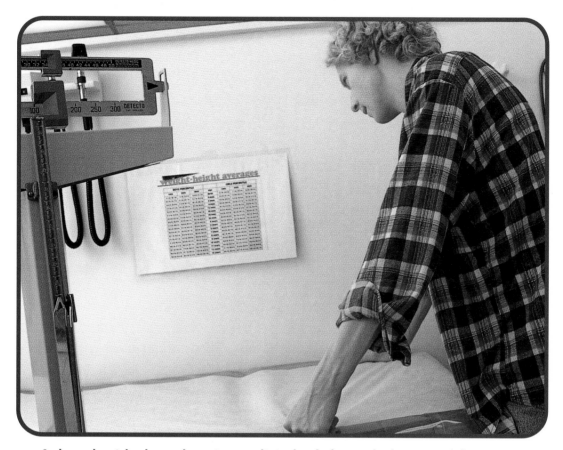

Scales and weight charts alone give us a limited and often misleading picture of a person's health.

that our bodies are genetically programmed to be a certain size or a specific weight: No matter how often you exercise or how many calories you count, your body fights to maintain its natural weight.

Our genes also influence our metabolism. Metabolism is the bodily process that determines how much of the fat in our food is turned into energy and how much is stored. Current research shows that our metabolism is also largely determined by our genes. This means that two people can eat the

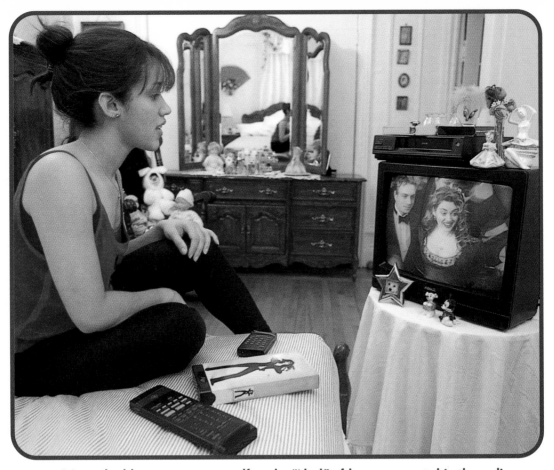

It's not healthy to compare yourself to the "ideal" of beauty presented in the media. Doing so could lead to a poor body image, depression, and eating disorders.

same amount of food, but one person will gain weight and the other will not. Weight differences occur because some people's bodies burn calories more slowly, not because they eat too much.

Comparing yourself to a cultural ideal can be dangerous to your health. Trying to be something that is unhealthy and unnatural for your body can lead to negative feelings about your body, which may lead to depression or result in a more serious eating disorder.

Jeanna

I am at the end of my rope. I have tried to diet, and I still look like a cow. Today I went to the drugstore and bought some diet pills and some laxatives. I read in a magazine that some people use them to lose weight. The pill box says that I won't feel hungry anymore if I take two pills before each meal. I am always hungry. Is this too good to be true? I don't know what to do. I wish I could talk to someone but nobody understands how awful I feel. Nobody knows what it's like to be me. I hate feeling fat.

Can you relate to Jeanna? We have all "felt" fat at some time. But fat is not a feeling, like happiness or fear. However, it's very common for people to attach feelings to food. Food, for many people, is not just fuel for their bodies. It's important to look at why food makes us feel certain ways so that we can change the way we look at food.

Food and Mood

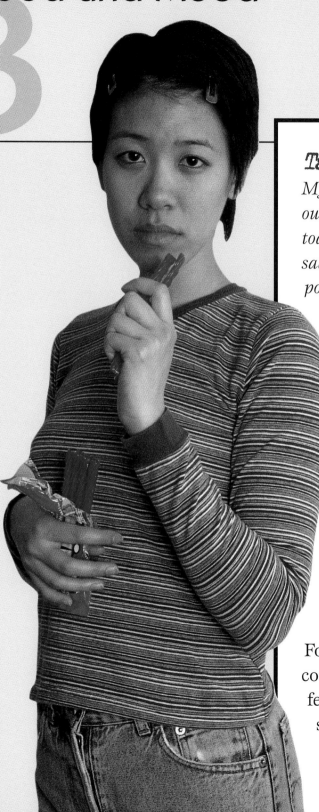

Tasha

My friends and I talked about our favorite comfort foods today at lunch. When I feel sad, I want salty food, like potato chips or french fries. My friend Sarah is crazy for cookies and candy. We all agree that chocolate can cure anything! I wonder why food makes us feel so much better.

Many people reach for something to eat when they feel upset. It is common to eat more when you feel under pressure or stressed out. Food somehow provides comfort in response to our feelings of anxiety, depression, sadness, or loss. Food is familiar and acceptable.

Food can fill up the emptiness inside us when we are feeling down.

You may have learned this behavior in childhood. Food is often used to reward children—a treat for being good or for a job well done. Wherever we learn our habits, food is used as a quick way to make ourselves feel better. But why?

Food and Feelings

The smell of apple pie at your grandmother's house . . . bacon and eggs cooking early in the morning . . . a table full of delicious food at every holiday. It's not unusual for food to become associated with certain feelings or memories. Certain foods make people feel safe and protected ("My mother always made me soup when I was sick." "Chocolate cake reminds me of the wonderful birthday parties I had when I was little."). Sometimes we crave or desire these foods for the feelings we have when we eat them.

Some people actually feel "good" or "bad" because of the foods they choose to eat. This is because they have assigned value to food—healthy food is "good" and junk food, or unhealthy food, is "bad." Choosing to eat only foods that are low in fat or low in calories makes people feel like they are strong or powerful and in control. This is a complicated issue, though: People may try to control their eating

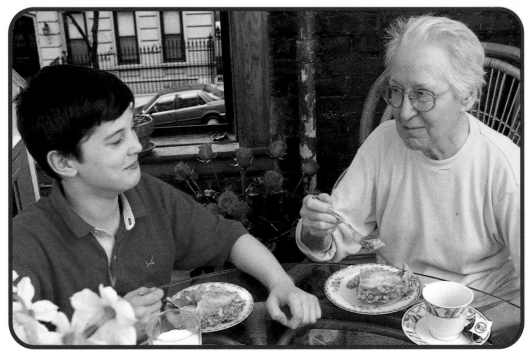

Sometimes we crave certain foods because of the good feelings and memories they trigger when we eat them. Often food is used as a way for friends and family members to bond.

because they feel that other parts of their lives are out of control, but they can control what they put in their mouths. They may consider others weak because they can't keep up with the strict rules of eating "good" food.

While eating healthy, low-fat food is smart, taking it to extremes can be unhealthy and even damaging. Fat is important for healthy, growing bodies. Too much fat is not good for anybody, but it's not the enemy, either. Fat actually tells your body when you've had enough to eat. If you don't eat enough fat, your brain won't know that you've had enough to eat, and you'll stay hungry.

Food Triggers

Most people may not realize that there is a lot of brain chemistry behind what we eat, when we eat, and why. Our diet influences the activity of nerve cells in our brains by activating chemical reactions. These chemical reactions affect the parts of our brain that control our behavior. Certain kinds of food trigger responses in our brains that make us feel happy, more relaxed, or more energetic.

Carbohydrates are one type of food that produces a dramatic emotional response in some people and are linked to specific brain chemistry. Many people, especially women, report a feeling of peace, calm, security, and even mild fatigue after eating large amounts of carbohydrates. Carbohydrates are the foods most commonly craved by people who overeat as a reaction to stress. Studies have found that carbohydrates actually affect the brain in the same way as some antidepressant medications prescribed by doctors. Unfortunately you can also experience a negative reaction and be overcome by a carbohydrate-produced fatigue—especially when you add to it the guilt about overeating.

From a sugar buzz to the sugar blues, people associate strong feelings and behaviors with eating sweet, sugary foods. In fact, many people believe sugar causes young children to be hyperactive.

There is no scientific evidence to support that claim, but there is plenty of research that shows that sugar can have a mood-altering effect. When you eat a food high in sugar, you experience an immediate rise in the level of sugar in your bloodstream, which feels like a quick boost of energy. Unfortunately, after the energy high comes an energy low—and your body works to control the level of sugar in your bloodstream. People commonly report being addicted to sugar, but doctors believe they are really hooked on the rush of energy they feel as a result of eating it. The relationship between food and feelings is not only emotional: scientific research shows it is a physical relationship as well.

Jeanna

I failed a test at school today. I know my mom is going to be so mad at me. I am really nervous about telling her. When I got home from school, I went to the kitchen for a snack, and before I knew it I had eaten a whole box of doughnuts. I can't even imagine all the fat and calories I just swallowed. I felt really good while I was eating. I forgot all about the test. But now my stomach hurts and I feel sick. I want to make myself throw up. Not only am I stupid, but I'm fat, too. I did not deserve to eat those doughnuts. I don't know what I was thinking.

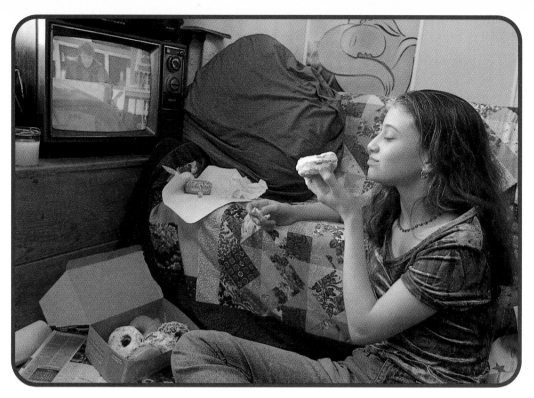

Drastically cutting back on the number of calories you consume puts your body into starvation mode. This can lead to a food obsession and episodes of bingeing.

The Cost of Dieting

Extreme dieting can be a painful process. Some doctors believe that people experience severe mood swings and depression as a result of strict diets. Studies have been conducted on dieters who take radical steps to cut calories and reduce food intake. More than half reported feeling nervous, weak, depressed, and anxious. People on strict diets actually send their bodies into a starvation mode.

If you "break" your diet because you suddenly can't resist high-fat or high-calorie foods, it is not necessarily a sign of weakness or lack of self-control. Your body could be pushing you to replenish its necessary supply of fats in the quickest, easiest way—by eating lots of fat. This is just one way your body may react when sent into a starvation mode.

Additionally, low-calorie diets that allow only a few types of foods can be bad for your health because they don't provide enough vitamins and minerals. Rapid weight loss from very low-calorie "starvation diets" can cause serious side effects in teenagers, such as gallstones, hair loss, weakness, and diarrhea.

Dieting may actually cause you to gain weight. Each time you sharply restrict your calorie intake, your metabolic rate slows down. When your metabolism slows down, your body burns fewer calories. This is because your body is trying to hold on to the little food it's getting. The body reacts to dieting by storing fat more efficiently in order to survive. When you stop dieting and increase your caloric intake, more weight is gained because your body stores more fat. Doctors warn against "yo-yo" dieting (repeatedly going on and off diets, losing and then gaining weight) because it can permanently affect your metabolism.

Dieters may report feeling high and "on top of the world" at the start of a diet. But these positive feelings quickly give way to depression and irritability. Dieters find themselves thinking and talking about all the food they are denying themselves. This can then lead to a diet-induced depression.

Breaking the Food/Mood Cycle

Think about all the ways you use food—to stop boredom, to socialize with friends, to give pleasure, or to mask pain. You can even make a list of how you use food. Now think about other things that might serve the same function as food. For instance, could you see a movie or go for a bike ride when you're bored, instead of eating? You may feel that nothing can replace the satisfaction you get from food, but it's important to come up with other options. You can learn how to make choices that will result in feeling better—either because you stop punishing yourself for eating or because you find a substitute activity. It might also help to identify situations that lead to overeating or a food craving. Identifying these situations can help you either avoid them or plan how to handle them.

You will be more successful in breaking the food/mood cycle if you can figure out what's really going on. What is the emptiness you are trying to fill—is it hunger or something more?

4

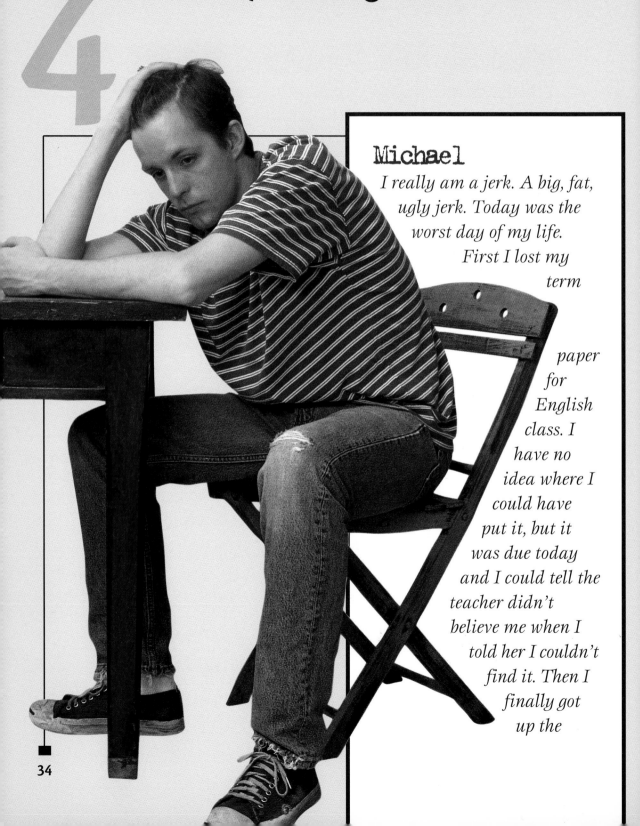

Michael

I really am a jerk. A big, fat, ugly jerk. Today was the worst day of my life. First I lost my term

paper for English class. I have no idea where I could have put it, but it was due today and I could tell the teacher didn't believe me when I told her I couldn't find it. Then I finally got up the courage to ask Amy out for Friday night. She looked at me as if I were speaking another language. If that's not bad enough, I spilled a soda in the cafeteria and got yelled at by Mr. Roberts in front of everyone. I wanted to fall through the floor when everyone laughed at me. I'm sure they were thinking I deserve all the bad luck for being such a fat slob. I hate looking like this!

As you can see from Michael's journal entry, he had a really lousy day. From the outside looking in, it seems to us that Michael's problems have to do with more than his weight or his appearance. So why is Michael so fixated on his looks as the root of his problems?

Without knowing it, Michael has fallen into a trap that is common among people with low self-esteem. Each of us has ongoing internal conversations with ourselves. These conversations are the way we sort out our thoughts and our perceptions of the world. We have these conversations without even consciously thinking about it, because it is a well-learned, unconscious habit. This makes it a very difficult habit to change.

Your Inner Critic

Michael's internal discussion is being dominated by the voice of his inner critic. Your inner critic is the voice inside you that speaks to you whenever you make a mistake or have bad luck; it is the voice that blames you for every misstep or misfortune, the voice that says you are never good enough. Unfortunately, most of us judge ourselves much more harshly than our peers do and we say things to ourselves that we would never accept from others.

The problem for people with low self-esteem is that they have accepted the voice of their inner critic as the voice of reality. If we let it, the inner critic will reinforce all the negative thoughts we have about ourselves and even create new worries and insecurities. Words like *fat* and *ugly* have become code words for Michael, and many other people. Michael feels embarrassed that he lost his homework, humiliated that he got in trouble and was turned down for a date: Those emotions feel like *fat* and *ugly* in Michael's head.

It doesn't matter to Michael if his weight is perfectly healthy. It doesn't matter if Amy actually likes him and thinks he's cute. As long as Michael feels fat and ugly, he will act as if he is. He has listened to his inner critic for so long, he doesn't question or challenge his belief that he is ugly and fat.

The first step toward creating a more positive body image is learning a new way of talking to yourself. To become aware of your inner conversation, start listening. What are you saying to yourself, about yourself—especially about your physical appearance?

What are you really feeling or experiencing when you say that you feel ugly? Record the comments of your inner critic in a journal as you start to change the tone of your internal discussion and develop your new, positive inner voice.

Real vs. Imagined Problems

Tasha

I had my annual checkup yesterday. Ugh! I hate going to the doctor. I'm always so scared that she'll tell me I am too fat and I need to go on a diet. She didn't weigh me, but we talked about my eating and exercise habits. She told me that dieting isn't healthy and I need to think about permanent lifestyle changes. She made a lot of sense. I guess I have some thinking to do.

Jeanna

I have lost seven pounds this week! What's even better is that I have been eating anything I wanted. I felt so sick after I ate all those doughnuts so I stuck my finger down my throat, and before I knew it, it was as if I had never eaten them in the first place. It was sort of gross—but I feel stronger and thinner already. Today Brian said hello to me in the hallway. He's never noticed me before. And Lucy and Mariana saved me a seat at lunch. I finally feel like I have some control over my weight and my life.

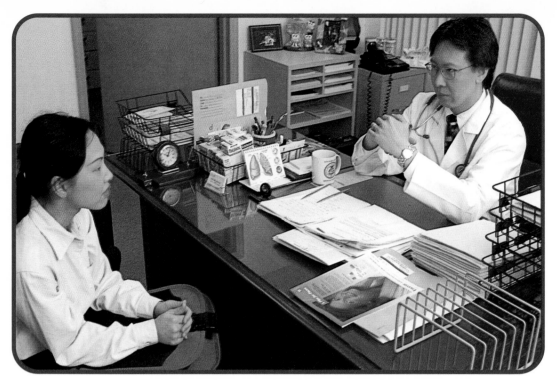

A doctor, or a registered dietitian, can help you change harmful attitudes about food and weight and teach you about healthy eating and exercise habits.

Many people believe they need to lose weight when, in fact, they are healthy just the way they are. But our society puts a lot of pressure on people to be thinner and "more beautiful," as we have discussed in previous chapters. Part of overcoming your body image issues is assessing whether you have a medical problem because your eating habits pose a risk to your health.

In order to help yourself and overcome your depression, it's important to make an effort to discover the true source of your negative self-esteem. This can be a very difficult thing to do. Our self-perception can be distorted after years of focusing on our flaws and imperfections. You may need the help of a counselor or therapist to help you discover the underlying factors behind your depression. You may think, "Well, the answer to changing my negative body image is to change my body!" It is understandable that most people wish to change their physical appearance as a way to feel better about themselves. However, improving our self-esteem and body image starts with accepting and loving ourselves for who we are, not how we look.

Fit at Every Size

Studies have shown that huge numbers of people who worry about their weight do not actually need to lose weight to be healthy. (You might think that it is impossible to be fit no matter what your body type.) More and more, though, doctors are emphasizing the need to be fit over the need to be thin. Many of the illnesses associated with being overweight are actually a product of inactivity. Regular exercise can improve your health more than losing weight. As we discussed in chapter 2, our size is, to some degree, beyond our control. Our genes determine what our behavior cannot change. This does not mean you can eat whatever you want and not worry about it. It does mean that good health is more than a number on a scale.

Eating Disorders

5

Jeanna

I feel great. The diet pills have really helped. I'm trying to watch what I eat, but sometimes I can't ignore my hunger. So when I ate a ton of cookies and half a gallon of ice cream, I made myself throw up. My mother finally said something to me—it took my losing twelve pounds before she even noticed. She is so busy with her own life, it's a miracle she even remembers I'm here. I thought about telling her, but I don't want to. It's nobody's business but my own. I went back to the drugstore instead of hanging out with everyone after school. I needed to buy more diet pills. I got some laxatives too. I just didn't feel like talking to everyone and watching them stuff their faces with junk from the vending machines. I just want to be alone.

While eating disorders most often affect females, an increasing number of males are also suffering. The reasons why a person develops an eating disorder are complex. They involve a person's eating habits, attitudes about weight and food, attitudes about body shape, and other psychological factors, such as depression. A person may be having problems in his or her family, job, school, or other relationships. A person may feel out of control in his or her life. Eating disorders are symptoms of these problems. Often, they are a way for people to take control over the one thing they can—their bodies.

Anorexia Nervosa and Bulimia Nervosa

Two of the most common eating disorders are anorexia nervosa and bulimia nervosa. Anorexia nervosa (often shortened to anorexia) is a dangerous eating disorder characterized by self-starvation. Even though people with anorexia may be extremely underweight, they see themselves as fat. They will resist all efforts to get them to eat or return to a

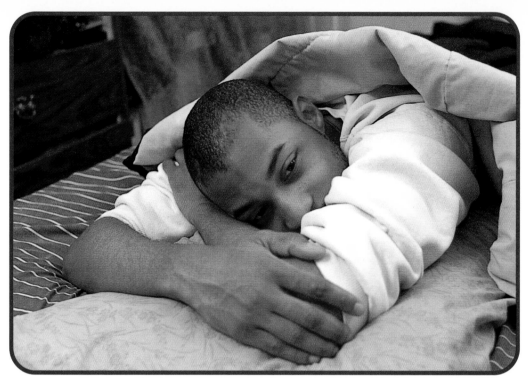

The number of males suffering from eating disorders is rising. Currently 1 million males in the United States struggle with anorexia, bulimia, and compulsive eating.

healthier weight. There are many dangerous physical and emotional results of anorexia.

People suffering from anorexia may show symptoms caused by severe weight loss: dry skin and hair, cold hands and feet, general weakness, constipation and digestive problems, insomnia (difficulty sleeping), and in women amenorrhea (loss of menstrual periods). As the weight loss progresses, more severe problems may develop, such as decreased resistance to infections, stress fractures, chemical imbalances, and weaknesses of the heart muscle that can lead to death.

Similar to anorexia, bulimia is fueled by an obsession with thinness and food. Bulimia (which means "ox hunger") is usually characterized by the overwhelming urge to binge and purge. People with bulimia engage in frequent, often daily, binge eating in which they consume very large amounts of food in a short time—mostly in secret. They then try to counteract the binge by purging the food from their body.

The methods of purging may include self-induced vomiting, abuse of laxatives and diuretics, enemas, diet pills, fasting, overexercising, or any combination of these. People with bulimia feel out of control and are victims to the cycle of bingeing and purging. They suffer from medical problems caused by the purging methods as well as their eating habits. Medical problems include dehydration, constipation and digestive disorders, severe dental problems, and muscle weakness. As bulimia progresses, ulcers and life-threatening heart irregularities may develop.

If You Think You Have an Eating Disorder

The most important thing to remember is that you are not alone and help is available to you. Eating disorders can be prevented: You can stop them before they start or you can keep them from becoming worse or recurring. If you think you have a problem, please consider getting help. Recovery is a difficult process, but many people do recover from eating disorders.

The first thing you should do is talk to someone. You might choose to talk to friends and family for the

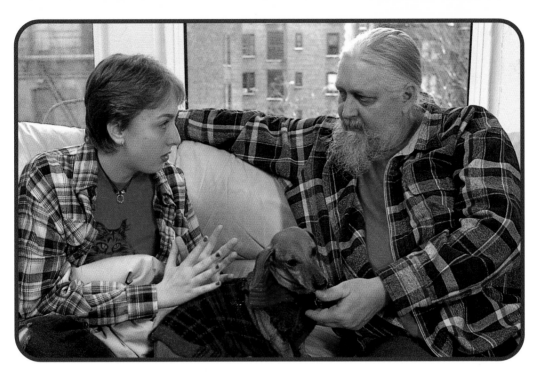

The first step toward recovery from an eating disorder is to share your problem with a trusted friend or adult who can offer support and guidance.

support and understanding they can provide. If they are available, you might choose a teacher, a guidance counselor, or someone from your church who can give you the support of an objective adult. These people can help you prepare for the emotional experience of sharing your secret with your family. You might also want to talk to a therapist, someone who is trained to help with eating disorders. Whomever you talk to, be sure it's someone you can trust. It's very important to be honest with that person so that he or she can accurately assess your situation and help you in the way that's best for you. Reaching out to someone and asking for help is a courageous step toward recovery.

The second step is to get more information. Call a help line, consult with a doctor, read a book on eating disorders, research Web sites on the Internet. Knowledge is power, and your goal is to take power back from the destructive habits and behaviors of your eating disorder. These resources will help you understand your eating disorder, share stories of others who have suffered from similar disorders, and help you work toward regaining your health and happiness.

Jeanna

Unbelievable! Lucy and Mariana told me at lunch that they wanted to talk to me privately after school today. I figured they wanted to hear about my diet, find out my secrets for success now that I have lost over twenty pounds. So I went to Lucy's house with Mariana, only to find that they wanted to tell me that I look terrible. They think something is wrong with me, that I am sick. I just sat there listening while they went on and on. I was furious. I know they're just jealous. I can't get fat: That's exactly what Lucy and Mariana want.

When a Family Member or a Friend Has an Eating Disorder...

If you think a friend or a family member has an eating disorder, there are things you can do to help. These topics are not easy to discuss. Here are some helpful suggestions:

1. Discuss your concerns with a professional. Learn about eating disorders and available local resources. Write or phone organizations (see Where to Go for Help) for printed material and lists of support groups in your area.

2. Talk to your friend. Keep the conversation informal and confidential, and focus your concerns on your friend's health, not weight and appearance. Explain how the problem is affecting your relationship. Mention that eating disorders can be treated successfully. If your friend can acknowledge the problem, suggest some resources.

3. Realize that you may be rejected. People with eating disorders often deny their problem because they're afraid to admit they are out of control. Don't take the rejection personally. Try to end the conversation in a way that will allow you to come back to the subject at another time.

4. Know your limits. If you sense that you're getting angry or impatient,

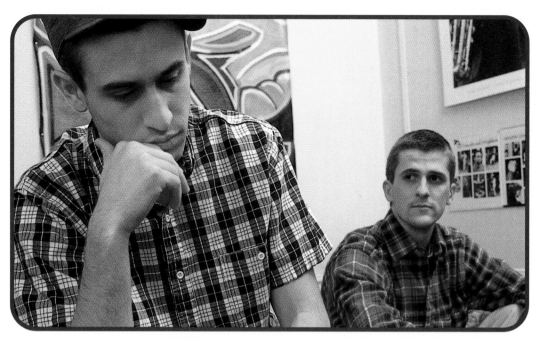

You can help a friend or a family member with an eating disorder by discussing your concerns with them in a supportive way. It's important to remember, however, that you cannot force anyone into treatment.

back off. Don't take on the role of counselor or food monitor—it's not your job and you're not qualified to do it. You might attend a support group to help you deal with your own pain and get advice on how to interact with your friend or family member.

5. Don't nag or bully. You can't recover for someone else. Be supportive in constructive ways. Offer to accompany your friend to therapy appointments, or express concern and interest in your friend's progress.

How to Help Yourself

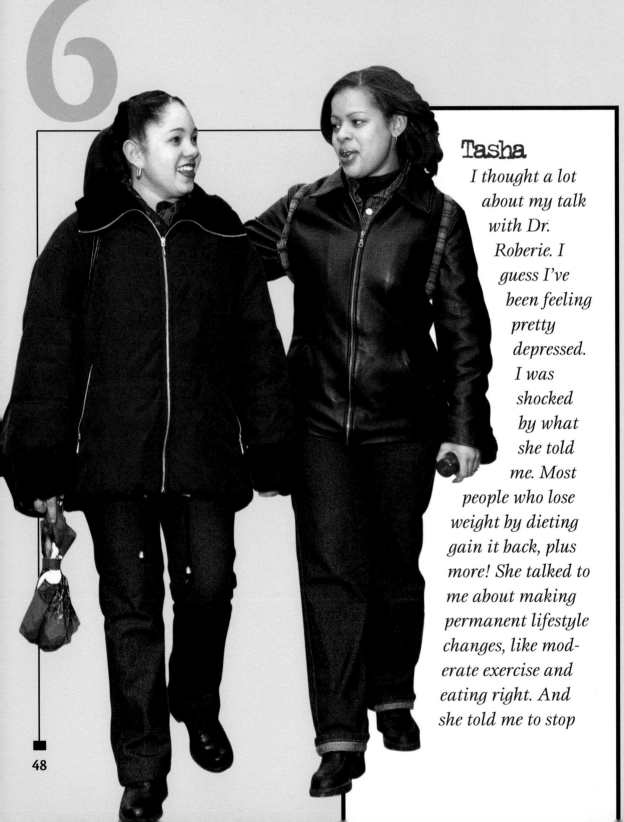

6

Tasha

I thought a lot about my talk with Dr. Roberie. I guess I've been feeling pretty depressed. I was shocked by what she told me. Most people who lose weight by dieting gain it back, plus more! She talked to me about making permanent lifestyle changes, like moderate exercise and eating right. And she told me to stop thinking about my weight and think about my health. I'm really worried, though. I love food—am I promising never to eat sweets? I think I'll try exercising. I have a friend who says she'll go walking with me after school. And I told my mother that I would walk the dog in the morning. Maybe that will help me feel better.

Tasha is on the right track. Making lifestyle choices that focus on her health, not her weight, will help her reach her goals. When people focus on losing weight and fail, they often give up on improving their health or engage in dangerous diet practices that may lead to eating disorders. Changing your attitude now can help you prevent this from happening.

The Benefits of Exercise

Exercise should be incorporated into every healthy person's life. Exercise is a great choice for Tasha and for many others as a starting point to changing one's body image. Tasha may not lose any weight from walking every day. But the emotional and mental gain will be worth her effort.

Medical research has proved that moderate amounts of exercise can reduce depression almost immediately. Exercise can also reduce tension, increase your energy, and improve your sleep. If you are feeling down for any reason, doctors recommend exercise as a simple, healthy way to combat depression. If you are feeling the body blues, you may receive even greater benefits from exercise. Not only will you experience reduced depression, but there is evidence that exercise promotes feelings of self-worth and personal confidence.

Changing Your Inner Critic

The key to helping yourself may be to change your thinking and your behavior. In the previous chapter, the suggestion to start keeping a journal of your feelings about yourself and your appearance is one example of a self-help exercise. The point of keeping a journal is to find the patterns in your self-criticism and to identify your inner critic. Do certain situations trigger your negative feelings? Do you focus on a certain part of your body? Identifying these patterns will help you develop your new inner voice—one that will drown out your old inner critic. Once you have things on paper, look for ways to challenge old assumptions. For example:

Old inner critic:
  "What I look like is an important part of who I am."

New inner voice:
  "How I behave and how I treat other people is an important part of who I am. My outer appearance is not a sign of my inner person. I am more than what I look like."

Old inner critic:

"The first thing people notice about me is what's wrong with the way I look."

New inner voice:

"The first thing people notice about me is my beautiful smile and how much fun it is to be around me."

Your new inner voice speaks the words you would like to believe. At first you may not believe these statements, but keep saying them. Make them a part of your everyday routine. This is a learned behavior, and it takes practice. It is also helpful to reward yourself for every small success.

Stop, Look, and Listen!

When you start feeling those body blues creeping up on you, practice a technique called "Stop, look, and listen." Stop your inner critic—even if you have to interrupt. Imagine a huge red STOP sign. Before you can change, you have to stop your negative thoughts cold. Look at or examine what you are thinking, saying to yourself, or feeling. What triggered your feelings? What are you feeling right now? What are you thinking that's making you feel so bad? Finally, listen to your new inner voice. It is there to challenge and dispute your old way of thinking. Take a couple of minutes to talk to yourself the way you would talk to a very good friend who has just said something mean about himself or herself.

Tasha

I feel a lot better this week. I have been taking a walk each evening, and sometimes I take a walk after school as well. I have been using the new diary my mom bought for me, and it feels good to get all my feelings out. I don't think I have been honest with myself for a long time. I checked a book out of the library on improving self-esteem. I started reading it last night. It looks okay, like maybe I will learn some helpful things.

Fat ! So?

Fat!So? is the name of an independent publication that battles to put an end to fat stereotypes. Activist movements in our country work to challenge society's thinking about fat. There are zines, books, newsletters, and magazines that promote the idea that all body shapes are beautiful. These movements are responsible for producing the new fashion magazine *Mode* for women sizes 12 and up, and for persuading stores to carry hip clothes in larger sizes.

You are a consumer and should feel free to write letters and make phone calls when you think you see or experience an example of fat discrimination. Many people find that fighting back against society's stereotypes and unreal ideals about how we should

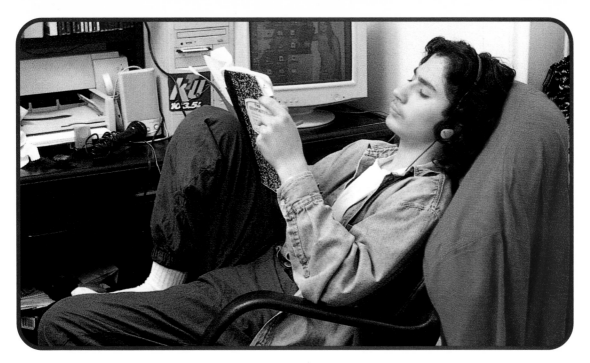

Teens need to be aware of the contant stream of messages they receive from the media—from television to movies to music. Taking a stand against negative images and messages will give you more self-confidence and a strong sense of purpose.

look helps them change their own ideals. Acting out and fighting back can provide a release for all those negative thoughts.

Tasha

I threw my scale away today. Who needs it? All it did was make me feel depressed. I can't believe I weighed myself every morning. No wonder I felt so terrible. Well, no more. I don't have time for that—I have a life to lead.

What Do You Do When You Need More Help?

There are numerous professionals who can guide you and support you in changing your body image and improving your self-esteem. You can choose which is the best and most comfortable fit for your specific needs. It is extremely important to choose someone you trust and someone who will work with you in partnership. Change is an active process that demands your commitment and participation.

You might choose to see a medical doctor or a psychiatrist. Both are licensed to prescribe medication, such as antidepressants, and can be helpful if you have a physical health concern. You could also work with a psychologist or a trained social worker. Neither can prescribe medication, but they are skilled professionals who can help you deal with emotional and psychological issues.

You might want to work with a team of professionals who provide a combination of different training and experience. The therapist you choose must be a person with whom you can be honest. The process and success of therapy depends on an honest, trusting relationship between the therapist and client.

Group and Family Therapy

In group therapy, each person shares his or her story, works with the group to find common solutions, and provides support for others. Another therapy option is to involve your family members in the meetings between you and your therapist. This is called family therapy. You might decide that you

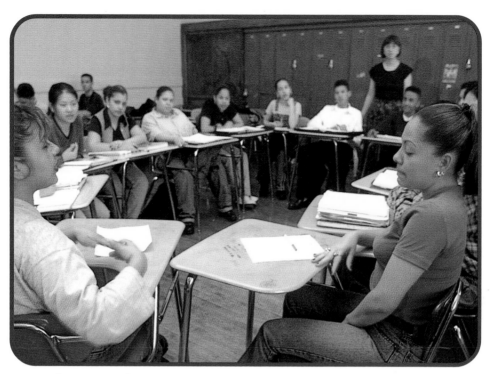

Group therapy provides a supportive environment in which you can share your experiences with others who have similar concerns. Realizing that you are not alone with your problems will help you improve your self-image.

need the support and understanding of your family in order to make permanent changes in your life. Often, young people feel that a certain pattern of behavior in their family contributes to their negative feelings. Talking to your parents in the presence of a therapist can help create a space where you can be honest with yourself and honest and open with your family.

Michael

I'm going to see a counselor today after school. I'm really nervous about it, but I've been feeling so low, I'm willing to try anything at this point. My mom is taking me, but I am talking to him alone. I don't know what I am going to say. I just realized there wasn't anyone else I could talk to. I am afraid my friends would laugh if I tried to talk to them, and I don't think my mom would understand. I guess it won't hurt to try talking to a therapist. Maybe it will even help.

Depending on how you want to implement change in your life, you might benefit from consulting a registered dietitian in addition to meeting with a therapist. A dietitian can provide accurate information about food and nutrition and help you plan meals and eating strategies. Choose someone who is registered, which means that he or she has received training and testing. A dietitian can help you work to accomplish your goals in a healthy and realistic way.

Now that you've read this book and have all this new information, what does it mean? What will you do next? Whatever you decide, reading this book has been a first step toward understanding yourself better and increasing your self-esteem—two important ingredients for a happy, successful life. The body blues is not a permanent condition. You have the power already within you to change your feelings, your actions, and your thoughts. Learning to accept yourself can be a lifelong journey—one well worth taking.

Glossary

activist Someone who gets involved to support or fight against a controversial issue.

addiction An uncontrollable need for and use of a substance or a behavior.

amenorrhea When a girl stops getting her period.

binge To consume large amounts of food, often in secret and usually without control.

carbohydrate An essential nutrient found in sugars, starches, grains, beans, fruits, and vegetables.

compulsion An irresistible impulse to perform an irrational act.

crave To have a strong desire for something.

culture Beliefs, accomplishments, and behavior patterns of a community or population, passed on from one generation to another.

depression A state of extreme and prolonged sadness.

dietitian A person trained in the field of nutrition and health.

diuretics Drugs that increase the flow of urine.

genes/genetic Qualities or tendencies that we are born with.

metabolism The process by which the body turns food into energy.

obsession Something you cannot stop thinking or worrying about.

psychiatrist A doctor who is trained to treat people with mental, emotional, or behavioral disorders.

purge To get rid of food suddenly and harshly, usually by vomiting, exercise, or laxatives.

self-esteem Confidence, self-respect, and satisfaction with oneself.

therapist A person trained in treatment of emotional disorders.

Where to Go for Help

American Dietitic Assocation
216 West Jackson Boulevard, Suite 805
Chicago, IL 60606
(312) 899-0040
Nutrition hotline: (800) 366-1655
Web site: http://www.eatright.org

Anorexia Nervosa and Related Eating Disorders, Inc. (ANRED)
P.O. Box 5102
Eugene, OR 97405
(541) 344-1144
Web site: http://www.anred.com

Eating Disorders Awareness and Prevention (EDAP)
603 Stewart Street, Suite 803
Seattle, WA 98101
(206) 382-3587
Web site: http://members.aol.com/edapinc

Mental Health Information Center
National Mental Health Association
1021 Prince Street
Alexandria, VA 22314-2971
(800) 969-NMHA
Web site: http://www.nmha.org

National Association of Anorexia Nervosa
and Associated Disorders (ANAD)
Box 7
Highland Park, IL 60035
(847) 831-3438
Web site: http://members.aol.com/anad20/
index.html

Overeaters Anonymous
Box 92870
Los Angeles, CA 90009
(800) 743-8703
Web site: http://www.overeatersanonymous.org

P.L.E.A.S.E. (Promoting Legislation and
Education About Self-Esteem)
91 South Main Street
West Hartford, Connecticut 06107
(860) 521-2515
e-mail: PLEASEINC@AOL.COM

In Canada

Anorexia Nervosa and Associated Disorders (ANAD)
109-2040 West 12th Avenue
Vancouver, BC V6J 2G2
(604) 739-2070

Web Sites:

If you have a computer and Internet access, the World Wide Web can be a great source of information!

The Body Shop. A Web site dedicated to improving self-esteem and self-respect for all people. http://www.the-body-shop.com

gURL. An online zine for young women with a lot of good straight talk about body image. http://www.gurl.com/

Go, girl! magazine. An online fitness magazine full of positive information and images for young women. http://www.gogirlmag.com/

Bring the Noise. A poll and information about media images and self-esteem/body image. http://www.mightymedia.com/youth/new/noise.cfm

For Further Reading

Ayer, Eleanor. *Everything You Need to Know About Depression*. New York: The Rosen Publishing Group, 1994.

Cash, Thomas F., Ph.D. *What Do You See When You Look in the Mirror?* New York: Bantam Books, 1995.

Cooke, Kaz. *Real Gorgeous: The Truth About Body and Beauty*. New York: W.W. Norton, 1996.

Crook, Marion. *The Body Image Trap: Understanding and Rejecting Body Image Myths.* Vancouver: Self-Counsel Press, 1991.

————.*Looking Good: Teenagers and Eating Disorders*. Toronto: NC Press Ltd., 1992.

Emme, and Daniel Paisner. *True Beauty*. New York: G. P. Putnam's Sons, 1996.

Hutchinson, Germaine. *Transforming Body Image: Learning to Love the Body You Have.* Freedom, CA: The Crossing Press, 1985.

Kano, Susan. *Making Peace with Food: Freeing Yourself from the Diet/Weight Obsession.* Rev. ed. New York: HarperCollins, 1989.

Index

About the Author

Laura Weeldreyer works on public school reform at a nonprofit organization in Baltimore, Maryland. A former teacher, she adapted and directed *Beauty Secrets: The Politics of Appearance*, an original production. Ms. Weeldreyer devotes her time and energy to causes that affect young people.

Design And Layout by Christine Innamorato

Consulting Editor: Michele I. Drohan

Photo Credits
All photos by Maike Schulz